Natural Beauty Secrets

By Kimmy Gerred Nelson

In the early nineties was the first time that I ever thought about doing something about a wrinkle. I had heard about alpha hydroxyl and that the juice from fruits could be used as alpha hydroxy in it's natural state.

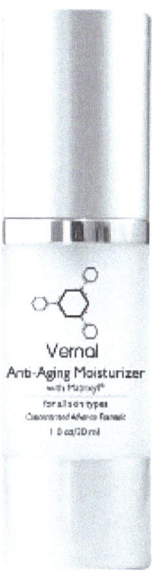

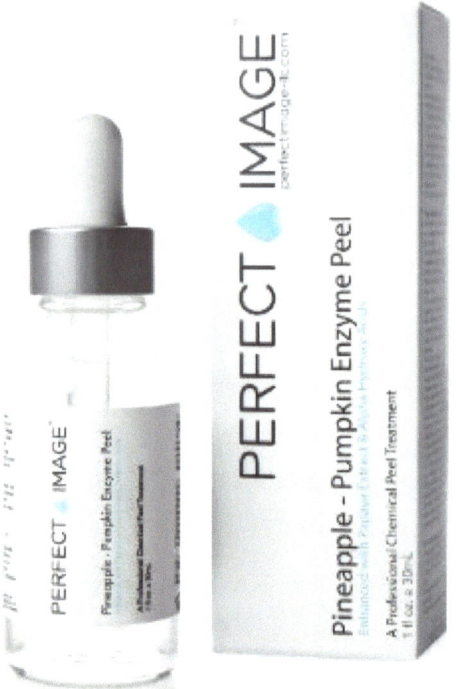

So I put a little fruit juice on a wrinkle and I rubbed it in a circular motion after my professor from "Anatomy & Physiology" had taught us that wrinkles were nothing more then the formation of dead cells.

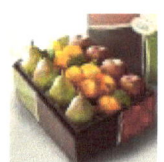

Almost the exact same cellular structure of dead cells that form our hair or finger nails. And that if you could get the old dead cells off of your face then the wrinkle would also vanish or greatly diminish. I tried it and it worked. It worked so well that I have used it ever since.

Only twenty years later my dermatologist found a spot on my shoulder and he removed it.

 Then he told me that I needed to stay [out of the sun](#) as much as possible or to use [sunscreen](#) all of the time when I am outside.

This "[Badger](#)" is an all natural sunscreen with 30 SPF. See a Photo of it on the next page as it would not fit on this page.

A lot of the products we list will be photo shot on the following page as the format will not allowed to go outside of the borders.

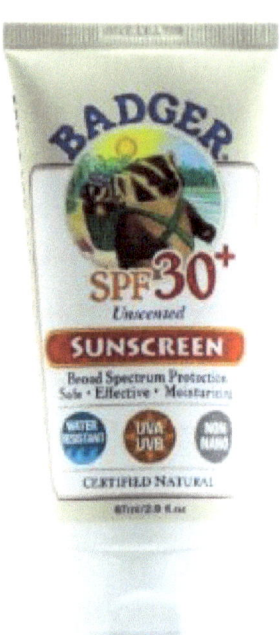

In college I took "Fashion & Clothing" too and I learned that there are a couple of things that really cause wrinkles more so then others. The sun causes wrinkles above all else. Secondly, wearing makeup to bed will also age your skin rapidly. Wear Shades!

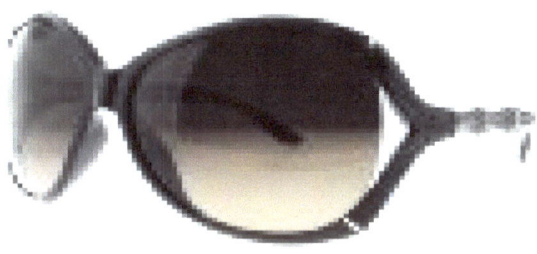

Some people don't like to wear sunscreen or they are simply allergic to it like me. I cannot drive if I put it on because my eyes water so much. So I recommend big sunglasses and a big hat for people who don't want to use sunscreen.

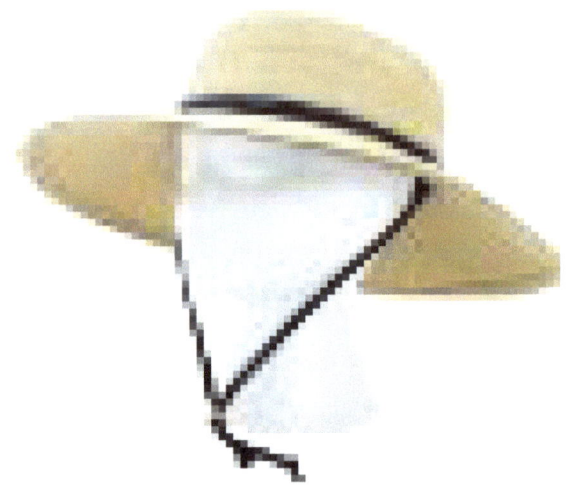

Thirdly, you want to stay away from products that contain mineral oil. I don't think it is wrong to use it on your [baby's skin](#) because that is what baby oil is. But I do not recommend it at all for anyone's hands for face if you want the skin to remain wrinkle free.

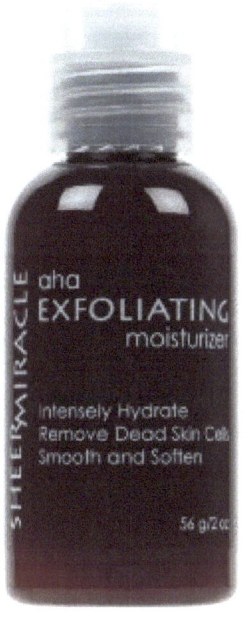

It was not too long after that when I turned on Trinity Broadcast Network and they had a Christian Dermatologist on some program and they were talking about skin protection.   He went on to talk about how to get rid of wrinkles by using alpha hydroxy and that it was important to use to use [sunscreen](). This one is my Favorite!

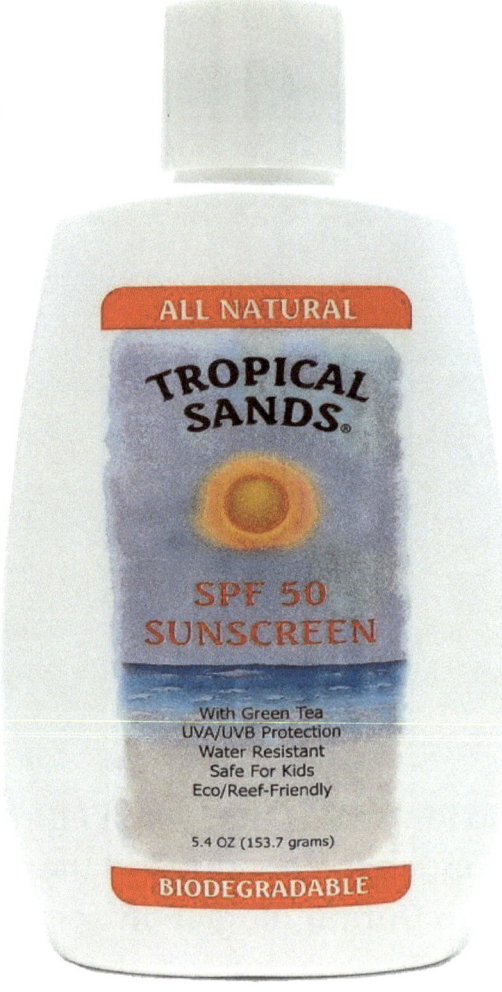

100% All Natural UVA/UVB Protection, Water Resistant, Safe For Kids, Eco/Reef Friendly, SPF 50! This is it!

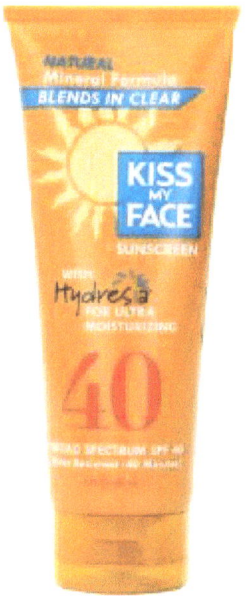

Here is another fine Sun Screen for the face.

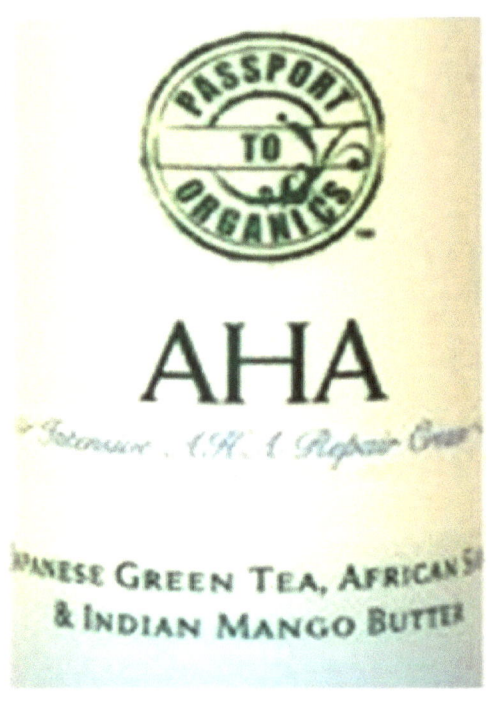

Anytime you use alpha hydroxy you must use sun screen to prevent further damage because now the skin will even be more

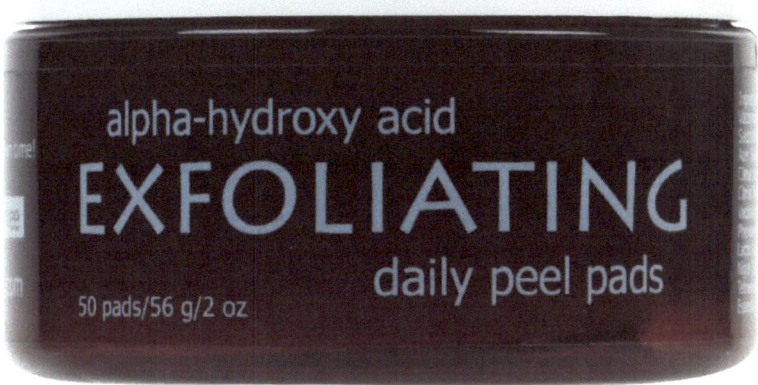

susceptible to the sun as the alpha hydroxy removes some of the top layer of skin.

He said that the best time to use the alpha hydroxy is at night time while we sleep. He said that was when it would be the most effective and the best time to use it if you were going to use it to fight wrinkles.

He also went on to tell us how important it is to use a moisturizer on your skin. He gave a simple recipe that I've been using every since. It is nothing more then simple safflower oil or coconut oil combined with raw sugar.

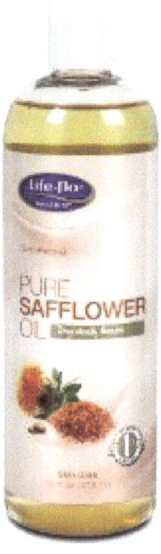

But I am not the kind of person who is going to go to sleep with raw sugar or sweet on my face because I don't want to attract bugs near my head when I am sleeping. And I found that the sugar and oil mixture is very sticky and the granules of sugar tend to fall off once they are dry and that only makes for a mess.

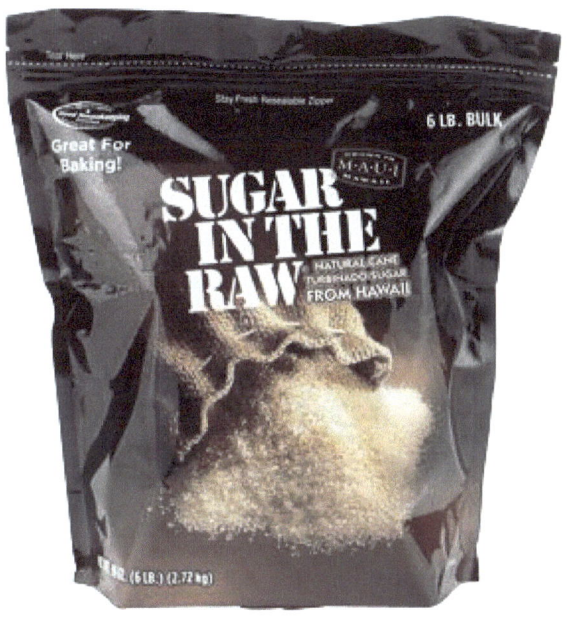

They make [alpha hydroxy](#) that you can buy and pay a lot of money for it. But I found that sugar and safflower oil work so much better and they certainly are more assessable and affordable.

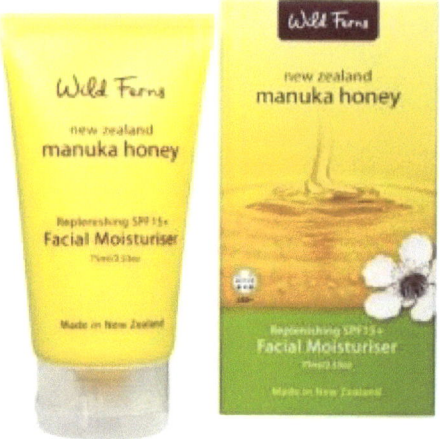

But you can accomplish the same wonderful effects of alpha hydroxy with some natural store bought products like moisturizers with honey in them. Or you could actually just use honey and safflower oil instead of sugar and safflower oil. At least that way it will not turn grainy and fall off. But it can still be too sticky.

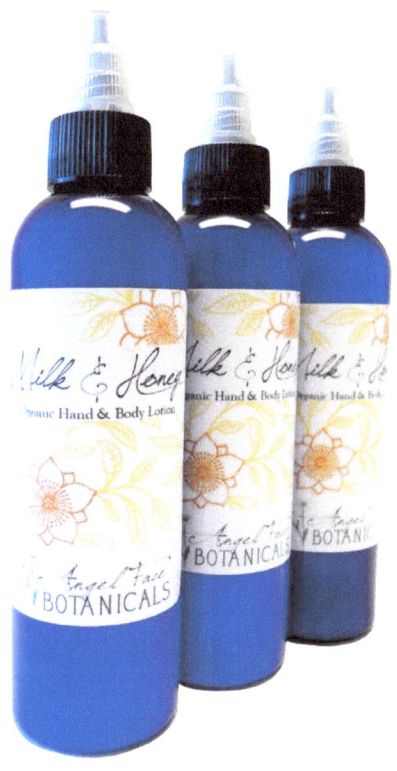

Next you will need to exfoliate on a weekly basis unless the alpha hydroxy that you use has it's own exfoliate in it which a few do.

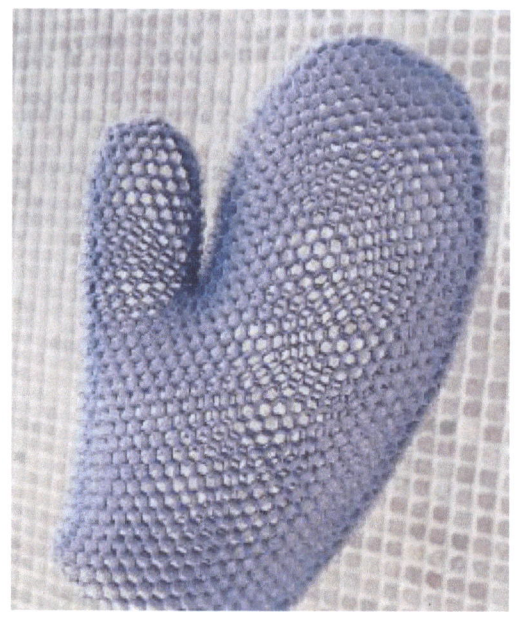

Personally, I use a hand mit loofa scrub once a week on my face. But you can also just use plain ole corn meal. Or you can try this Two Speed Rotating Facial Scrub Brush by Olay

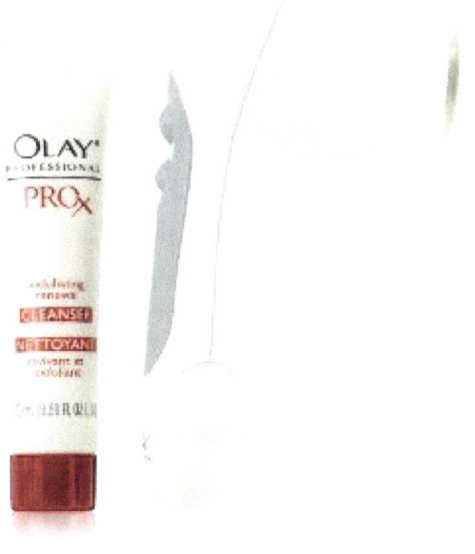

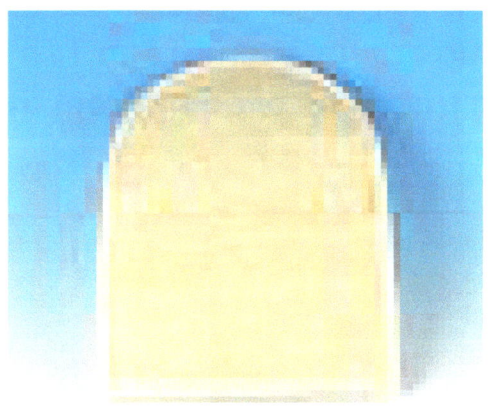

There was a time when I was instructed to just simply use plain ole corn meal and I did. It worked marvelously. And probably had some added benefits besides just removing the dead skin cells. Maybe it had some kind of mineral rejuvinator or anti oxidant effect. I just know it worked.

Red Rooibos always has great all natural skin benefits as it is trace minerals and vitamins in ample supply and it contains a nutrient found in the skin of an egg shell known as "hydroxy acid" or Alpha Hydrox.

Rooibos Tea contains zinc and alpha hydroxy acid which promote healthy skin. And because Rooibos has about fifty times more antioxidants then Green Tea it also reverses the signs of aging from the inside out.

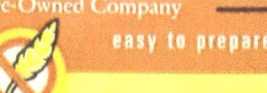

WHOLE
GRAIN
19g or more
per serving
EAT 16g OR MORE OF
WHOLE GRAINS DAILY

An Employee-Owned Company

moist and light   easy to prepare

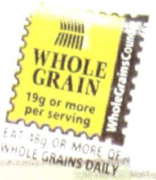

WHEAT FREE
GLUTEN FREE
DAIRY FREE

CORNBREAD MIX

ALL
NATURAL
PRODUCT

YOU CAN
SEE OUR
QUALITY

Bob's **Red Mill** ®

Stone ground whole grain cornmeal and sorghum impart an
unmatched flavor and texture from another era to our Gluten Free
Cornbread Mix. After easy preparation you will bake perfectly
moist and light cornbread.

Casein Free   NET WT 20 OZ (1 LB 4 OZ) 567g   K

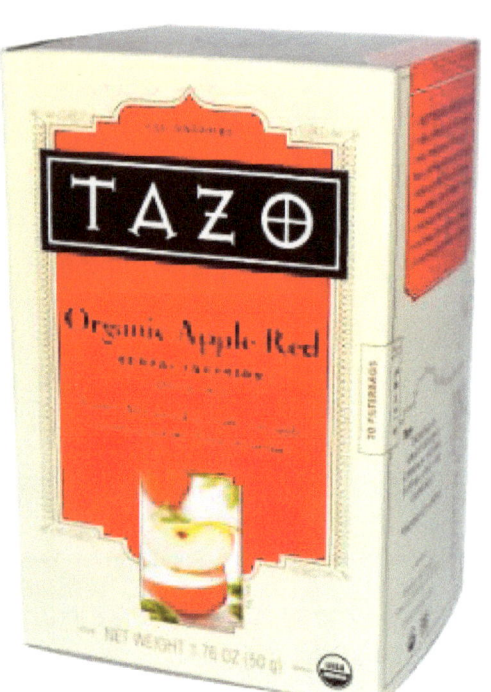

It is also important to have the right lifestyles and food choices that support a healthy skin foundation.

[Vitamin A & D](#) supplements in the oil softgels are great to take orally and to use topically in areas where wrinkles are likely.

That don't smell like roses unless you add a rose scent to cover it but I assure you that it is well worth it. Besides they make other supplements called "[Hope In A Jar](#)"

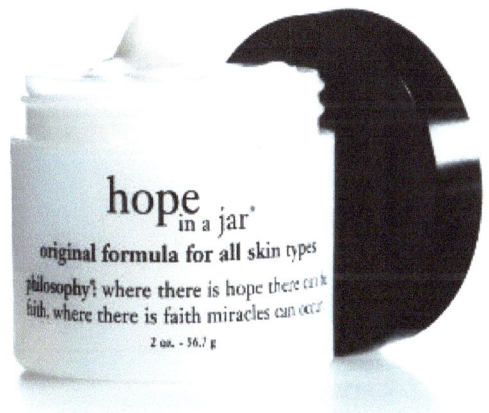

or Dianne Younger's facial serum that also have a different smell but the products work!

Here you will see [Orlane Crème Royale Neck and Decollete](#) though I cannot recall the scent of this one. It has remarkable results!

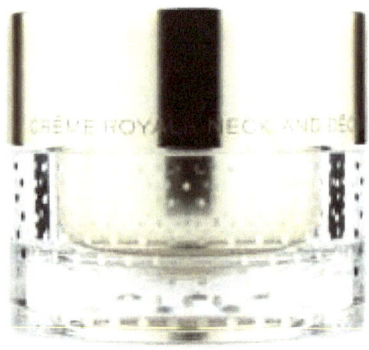

_____

The good thing with Vitamin A & D is that you can put on some scented safflower oil on top of it and it will cover the slight fresh sea scent of the Vitamin A & D.

DMAE is another supplement that has remarkable effects to improve skin appearance. Here you find the [DMAE & Arginine Firming Cream.](#) There are some products that acutally contain Rooibos Tea in the topical facial product and application too.

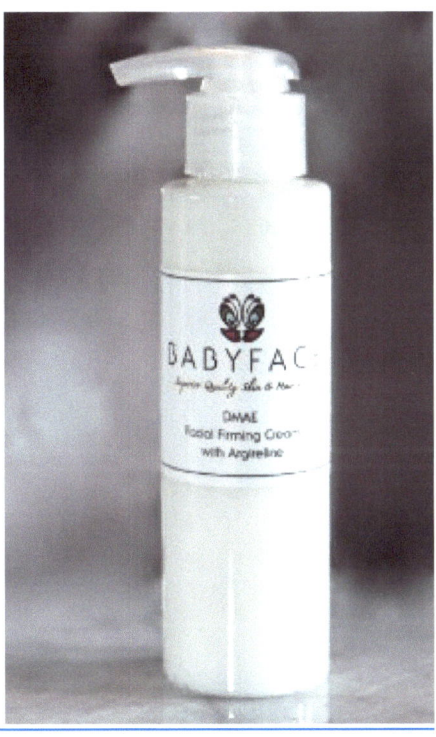

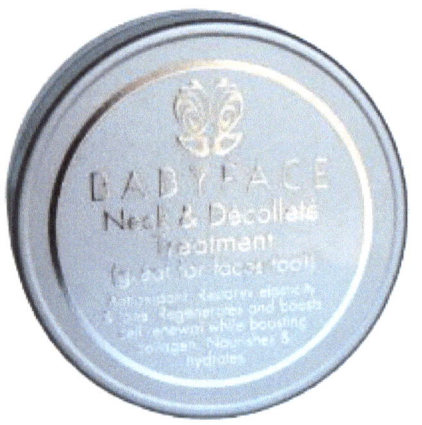

This Is BabyFace Face & Neck Cream with Antioxidants, Peptides, Hydration & Anti-Aging Royal Jelly, Bee Propolis, Argiline, Squaline, Coenzyme Q10, Retinol, Vitamin C

Here is Angel Face Rooibos and MSM Moisturizer

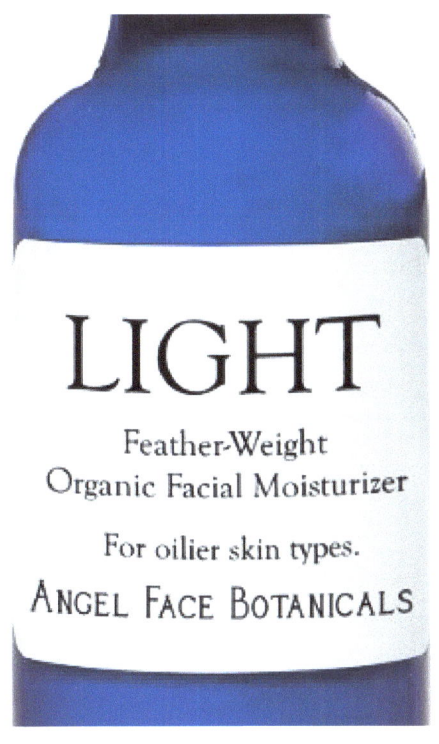

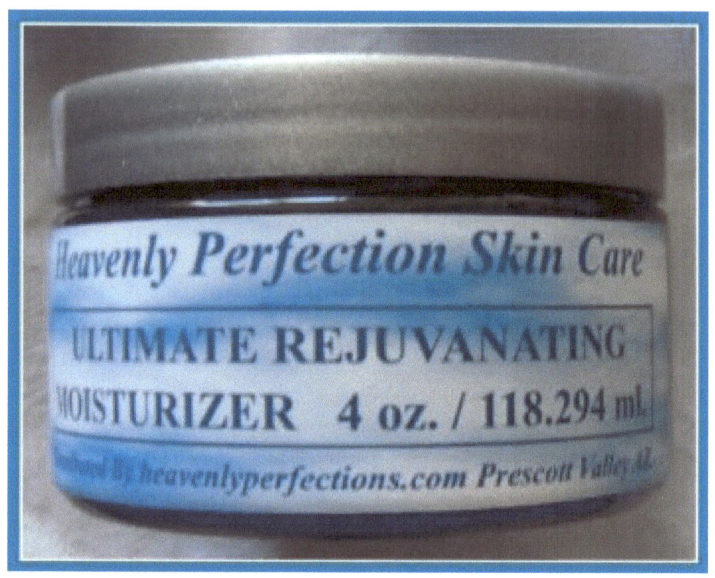

[This one is "Heavenly Perfection Skin Care" Ulitmate Rejunanating Moisturizer](#)

It is 81% Organic and contains DMAE, MSM, Rooibos, Pomegranate extracts and Hyaluronic Acid and at a very good price I might add. This is one of the best products that I've listed so far in terms of what you get and cost.

A milk facial is helpful when you need to restore the moisture and supple feel of soft skin. It is always good to have a box of instant milk on hand to bathe with occasionally too.

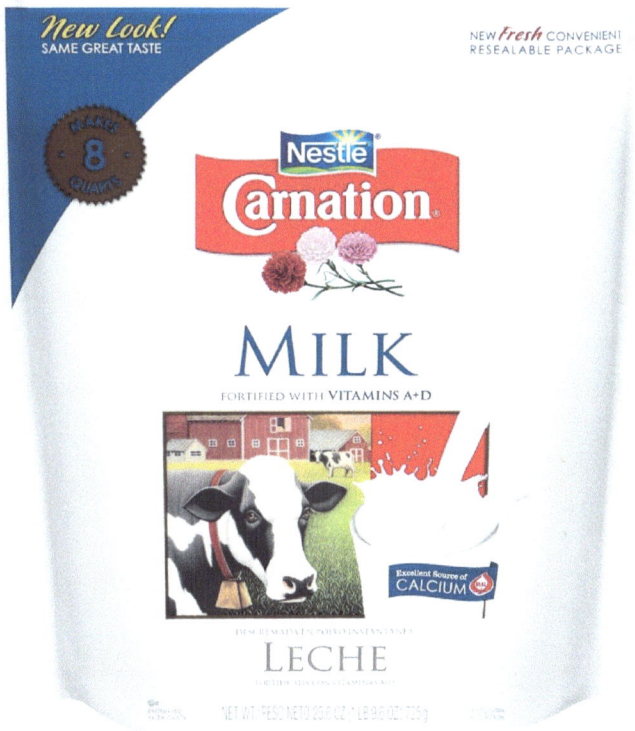

In the bath soak you just add about three cups of powdered milk to a whole large bath tub of water and soak in it for 15 minutes. Rinse off completely in a shower of warm water.

For a facial just apply milk directly to your face using a cotton ball. Leave it for fifteen minutes then rinse with water.

They also make [products with milk](#) in them so you don't have to do all the dirty work.

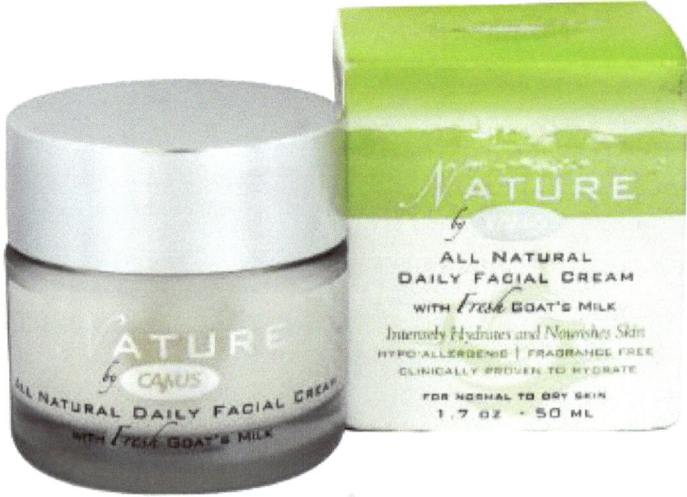

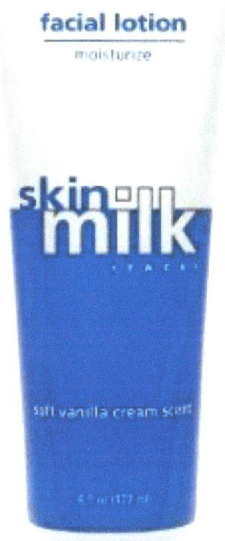

This Skin [Milk has Vanilla Scent](#) to it and makes it especially nice.

And some have sworn that mineral mud masks like "[Pure](#)" from the Dead Sea brought them renewed youth.

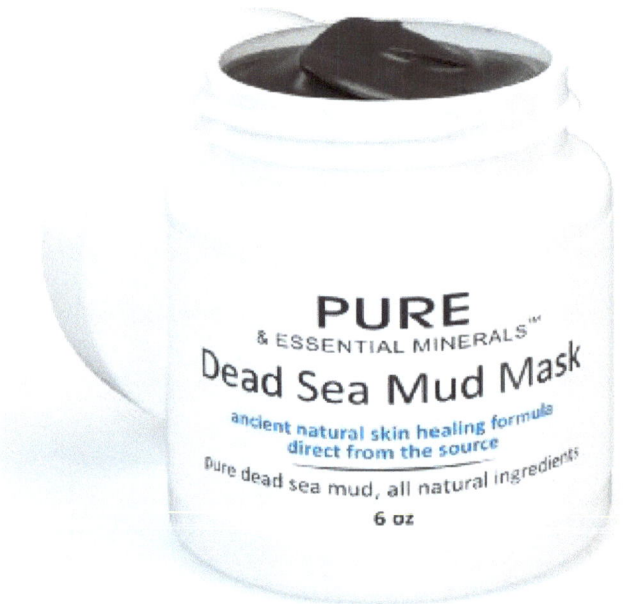

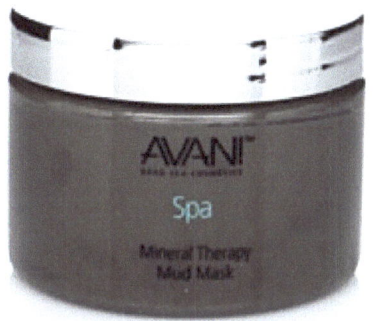

Or In [Avani Mineral Mud Mask](#) from the Dead Sea

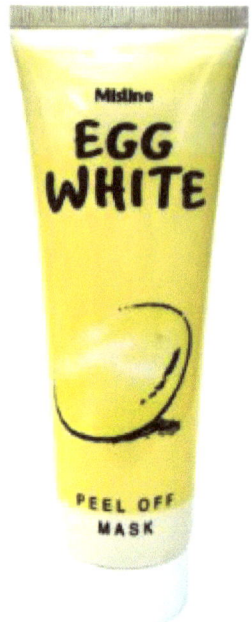

Eggs are particularly good to refine pores and tighten your skin. You can also find them already prepared in some facial products like "Egg White" Peel Off Mask.

Or like the Eggs In [SkinFood Egg White Mask](#) used to refine skin pores and tighten the skin like a face lift.

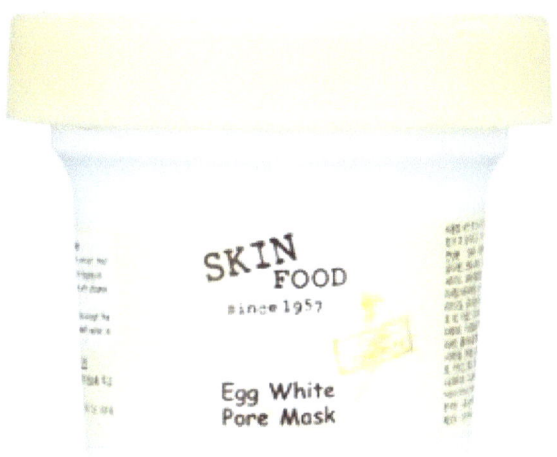

If you have a problem with eyes swelling as I do after I cry or if my nose gets stuffy then you can do as I do. I take Boswellia and Turmeric or Bromelain to stop the inflammation from the inside.

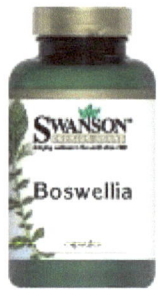

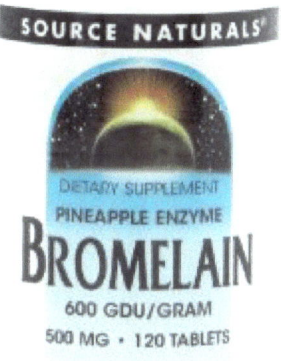

Bromelain stops swelling and inflammation. It is Pineapple Enzyme.

Taken on an empty stomach at the start of each day it can also prevent cancer. You can have water with it but don't eat for another thirty minutes.

Stop eye swelling instantly on the outside by using Hydrocortisone Cream (NOT OINTMENT)

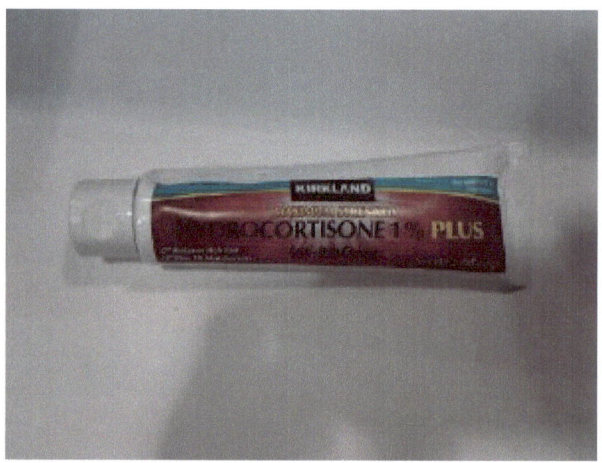

[Collagen](#) is really good for the skin. But if you are getting the right amount of Vitamin C every day then your body will produce it's own [collagen.](#)

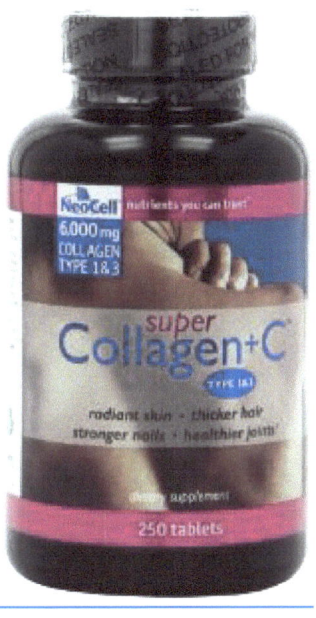

Here is some homeopathic scent of [Lavender](#) that you can add a drop or two to some safflower oil to use on top of the Vitamin A & D softgels once they are applied to the skin.

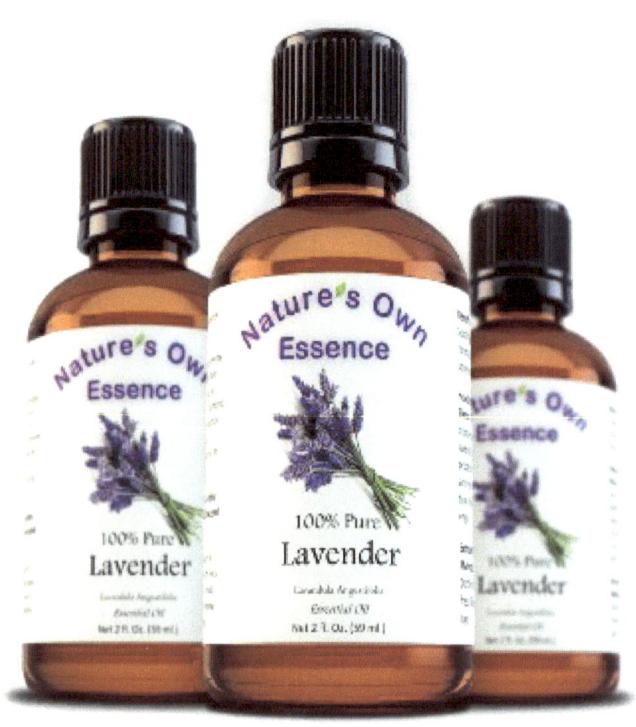

We hope that you find lots of healthy and natural ways to remain beautiful inside and out. Thank you!

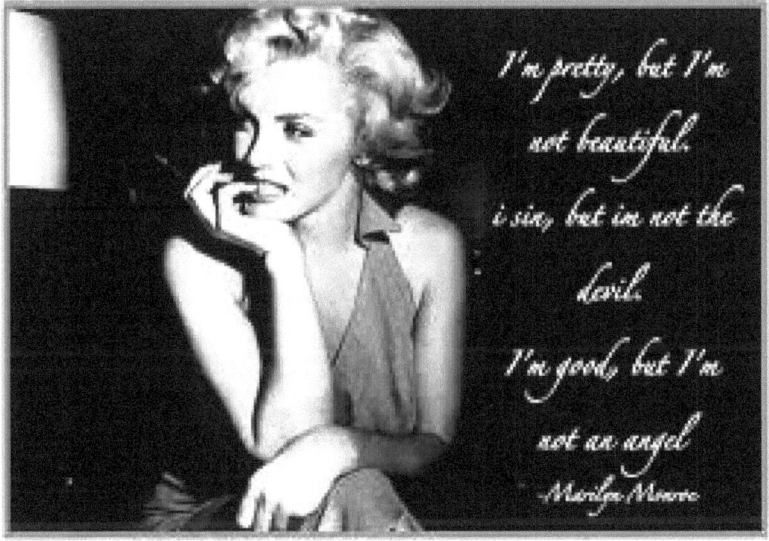